HEARING HEALTH 101

Unraveling the Mysteries of Hearing Loss and Methods for Sound Health

JENNIE BOSS

HEARING HEALTH 101

By Jennie Boss MD

February 2024

© Mind Heal Publishing

All Rights Reserved

CONTENTS

INTRODUCTION

Our ability to hear is fundamental to how we experience the world around us. From the laughter of loved ones to the melodies of music, sound enriches our lives in countless ways. However, hearing loss and related balance issues can pose significant challenges, affecting our relationships, work, and overall well-being. In this book, we shall embark on a journey to explore the intricate world of hearing health, unraveling the mysteries behind hearing loss, and discovering effective methods for maintaining sound health.

This book is designed to be a comprehensive guide, offering insights into the causes of hearing loss, preventive measures, and strategies for improving the quality of life for those affected by these conditions. Whether you are personally experiencing hearing loss or seeking to support a loved one, the information presented here aims to empower you with knowledge and practical solutions.

Let us embark on this journey together, as we research into the complexities of hearing health and uncover the keys to sound living. As we journey through these chapters, you will gain valuable insights and practical tools for nurturing your hearing health and enhancing your overall quality of life.

Jennie Boss MD

Page **8** of **103**

CHAPTER 1

THE WONDERS OF HEARING

The human auditory system is a marvel of biological engineering, allowing us to perceive and interpret the rich tapestry of sounds that surround us. From the gentle rustle of leaves to the concerto of voices in conversation, our ability to hear shapes our understanding of the world.

Anatomy of the Auditory System

At the heart of our ability to hear lies the complex structure of the auditory system. The process begins with the external ear, comprising the pinna (outer ear) and the ear canal, which funnel sound waves towards the eardrum.

Once sound waves reach the eardrum, they cause it to vibrate, transmitting these vibrations through three tiny bones in the middle ear: the malleus (hammer), incus (anvil), and stapes (stirrup). These bones amplify and transmit the vibrations to the cochlea, a spiral-shaped organ in the inner ear filled with fluid and lined with thousands of sensory hair cells.

As the fluid in the cochlea vibrates, it stimulates the hair cells to convert these vibrations into electrical signals, which are then transmitted via the auditory nerve to the brain for processing. Remarkably, this intricate process occurs within milliseconds, allowing us to perceive sound instantaneously.

Physiology of Hearing

The perception of sound involves a complex interplay of sensory pathways within the brain. The auditory cortex, located in the temporal lobe, is responsible for processing and interpreting auditory information received from the ears.

Sound is not merely a sequence of vibrations but a rich tapestry of frequencies, intensities, and timbres. Our auditory system can distinguish between subtle variations in pitch, allowing us to appreciate the nuances of music and language.

Authority Citations

1. According to the American Speech-Language-Hearing Association (ASHA), the auditory system

is a highly specialized sensory system that enables humans to perceive and interpret sound.

2. In their publication "Anatomy and Physiology of the Ear," the National Institute on Deafness and Other Communication Disorders (NIDCD) provides detailed insights into the intricate anatomy and function of the auditory system.

3. Dr. Albert Edge, a leading researcher in auditory science at Harvard Medical School, has contributed extensively to our understanding of hair cell regeneration and the mechanisms of hearing loss and restoration.

The wonders of hearing extend far beyond mere sound perception. It enriches our experiences, fosters communication, and connects us to the world around us. As we journey deeper into the mysteries of hearing, let us marvel at the intricacies of this remarkable sensory system and the profound impact it has on our lives.

CHAPTER 2

UNDERSTANDING HEARING LOSS

Hearing loss is a prevalent and multifaceted condition that can affect individuals of all ages and backgrounds. It can manifest in various forms, ranging from mild to profound, and a myriad of factors, both environmental and genetic, can cause it.

Types of Hearing Loss

There are three primary types of hearing loss:

1. Conductive Hearing Loss

This type of hearing loss occurs when there is a problem with the transmission of sound waves from the outer or middle ear to the inner ear. Common causes include ear infections, fluid accumulation, and abnormalities of the ear canal or middle ear bones.

2. Sensorineural Hearing Loss

Sensorineural hearing loss results from damage to the inner ear or the auditory nerve. This damage can be caused by aging, prolonged exposure to loud noise, genetic factors, ototoxic medications, and certain medical conditions.

3. Mixed Hearing Loss

Mixed hearing loss involves a combination of conductive and sensorineural components, affecting both the middle and inner ear. Causes may include chronic ear infections, trauma, or genetic predisposition.

Causes of Hearing Loss

The causes of hearing loss are diverse and can vary depending on the type and severity of the condition. Some common causes include:

1. Aging

Presbycusis, or age-related hearing loss, is a natural consequence of aging and typically affects high-frequency sounds.

2. Noise Exposure

Prolonged exposure to loud noise, such as machinery, concerts, or firearms, can damage the delicate structures of the inner ear.

3. Genetics

Certain genetic mutations and hereditary factors can predispose individuals to hearing loss from birth or later in life.

4. Medical Conditions

Chronic diseases such as diabetes, cardiovascular disorders, and autoimmune conditions can impact hearing health.

5. Ototoxic

Medications: Some medications, including certain antibiotics, chemotherapy drugs, and nonsteroidal anti-inflammatory drugs (NSAIDs), can damage the inner ear and cause hearing loss.

Prevalence of Hearing Loss

Hearing loss is a global public health concern, affecting individuals across all age groups and demographics. According to the World Health Organization (WHO), approximately 466 million people worldwide live with disabling hearing loss, with the prevalence expected to rise due to population aging and increased noise exposure.

Authority Citations

1. The World Health Organization (WHO) provides comprehensive data and statistics on the global burden of hearing loss and its impact on public health.

2. The National Institute on Deafness and Other Communication Disorders (NIDCD) conducts

research and disseminates information on hearing loss and related disorders.

3. Dr. Christine Petit, a renowned geneticist and neuroscientist at the Collège de France, has made significant contributions to our understanding of the genetic basis of hearing loss.

Understanding the types, causes, and prevalence of hearing loss is essential for early detection, intervention, and management. As we delve deeper into the complexities of hearing health, let us strive to raise awareness and promote access to comprehensive care for individuals affected by hearing loss.

CHAPTER 3

BALANCE AND EQUILIBRIUM

Balance is a fundamental aspect of human function, enabling us to maintain stability and orientation in our environment. Our sense of balance, also known as equilibrium, is intricately linked to the inner ear, where specialized structures play a crucial role in detecting and processing spatial information.

Anatomy of the Vestibular System

The vestibular system, located within the inner ear, consists of several interconnected structures responsible for detecting motion and orientation. These structures include:

1. Semicircular Canals:

Three fluid-filled tubes arranged perpendicular to each other, detecting rotational movements of the head in three-dimensional space.

2. Otolith Organs:

Comprising the utricle and saccule, these structures detect linear accelerations and changes in head position relative to gravity.

3. Vestibular Nerve:

Transmitting sensory information from the inner ear to the brainstem and vestibular nuclei, where it is processed and integrated with visual and proprioceptive inputs.

Functions of the Vestibular System

The vestibular system serves several critical functions in maintaining balance and equilibrium:

Spatial Orientation

Detecting changes in head position and orientation relative to gravity, allowing us to maintain upright posture and navigate our surroundings.

Dynamic Stability

Detecting and responding to motion, facilitating smooth movements and adjustments to changes in direction and velocity.

Visual Stabilization

Coordinating eye movements to stabilize visual images during head motion, ensuring clear and focused vision.

Disorders of Balance

Disruptions to the vestibular system can lead to balance disorders, causing symptoms such as dizziness, vertigo, and unsteadiness. Common balance disorders include:

1. Benign Paroxysmal Positional Vertigo (BPPV)

Characterized by brief episodes of vertigo triggered by changes in head position, often due to displaced calcium crystals within the inner ear.

2. Meniere's Disease:

A chronic condition characterized by recurrent episodes of vertigo, fluctuating hearing loss, tinnitus, and a sensation of fullness in the ear.

3. Vestibular Neuritis:

Inflammation of the vestibular nerve, leading to sudden onset of severe vertigo, nausea, and imbalance, often preceded by a viral infection.

Authority Citations

1. The Vestibular Disorders Association (VEDA) offers valuable resources and information on balance disorders, including diagnosis, treatment, and support services.

2. Dr. Michael Strupp, a leading neurologist and expert in vestibular disorders at Ludwig Maximilian

University of Munich, has contributed extensively to our understanding of the pathophysiology and management of balance disorders.

Understanding the anatomy and function of the vestibular system is essential for diagnosing and managing balance disorders effectively. As we delve deeper into the complexities of balance and equilibrium, let us strive to promote awareness, research, and access to care for individuals affected by vestibular dysfunction.

CHAPTER 4

EARLY SIGNS AND SYMPTOMS OF HEARING LOSS

Hearing loss is a condition that can manifest gradually, often with subtle signs and symptoms that may go unnoticed or ignored. Recognizing these early indicators is crucial for timely intervention and management of hearing loss to prevent further deterioration and mitigate its impact on quality of life.

Subtle Signs of Hearing Loss

Several subtle symptoms occur in a person to reveal hearing difficulty. These vary depending on the person's peculiar case. The following are some of these symptoms:

1. Difficulty Understanding Speech

Individuals may struggle to understand conversations especially in noisy environments. This may also happen when multiple people are speaking simultaneously. The patient struggles to understand what each person is saying or what the sound he hears means.

2. Frequent Asking for Repetition

Constantly asking others people to repeat what they said, or misunderstanding what they said can be an early indication of hearing impairment. A normal person with sound hearing will not habitually ask one to repeat himself or herself. When you see someone telling you, please, come again; it could be a sign of hearing challenge.

3. Increased Volume on Electronic Devices

Turning up the volume on televisions, radios, or smartphones to levels that others find uncomfortable may suggest difficulty hearing softer sounds. Do not confuse this with persons who naturally like noise even though it is not healthy for their ears. Yet, some persons reveal a situation of hearing difficulty when they often increase volumes on audio devices.

4. Withdrawal from Social Activities

Avoiding social gatherings or withdrawing from conversations due to difficulty hearing can be a sign of embarrassment or frustration associated with hearing loss. Such persons find it uncomfortable hanging around others who may not understand their condition.

5. Tinnitus

The perception of ringing, buzzing, or other phantom noises in the ears, known as tinnitus, is often associated with hearing loss and may indicate damage to the auditory system. When there are no such noises but someone hears them, probe the situation; it could be a hearing loss problem.

Risk Factors for Hearing Loss

Several factors increase the risk of developing hearing loss, including:

1. Age

Age-related hearing loss, known as presbycusis, is a common condition that affects many older adults due to natural changes in the auditory system over time.

2. Noise Exposure

Prolonged exposure to loud noises, such as occupational or recreational activities, can damage the delicate structures of the inner ear and lead to hearing loss.

3. Genetics

Family history of hearing loss or genetic predisposition may increase the likelihood of developing auditory impairment.

4. Medical Conditions

Certain medical conditions, including diabetes, cardiovascular disease, and autoimmune disorders, can impact hearing health and contribute to hearing loss.

5. Medications

Ototoxic medications, such as certain antibiotics, chemotherapy drugs, and nonsteroidal anti-inflammatory drugs (NSAIDs), can damage the auditory system and cause hearing loss.

Importance of Early Intervention

Early detection and intervention are critical for managing hearing loss effectively and minimizing its impact on daily life. Seeking prompt evaluation by a qualified audiologist or healthcare provider can facilitate timely diagnosis and access to appropriate treatment options, including hearing aids, assistive listening devices, and auditory rehabilitation programs.

Authority Citations

1. The American Academy of Audiology (AAA) emphasizes the importance of early detection and intervention for hearing loss to improve outcomes and quality of life for affected individuals.

2. The Hearing Loss Association of America (HLAA) provides resources and support for individuals with hearing loss and advocates for increased accessibility to hearing healthcare services.

Recognizing the early signs and risk factors for hearing loss empowers individuals to take proactive steps towards preserving their hearing health and seeking necessary interventions when needed. As we strive to raise awareness and promote hearing wellness, let us prioritize regular hearing screenings and embrace a proactive approach to auditory health.

CHAPTER 5

PREVENTION IS KEY

In the realm of hearing health, prevention plays a paramount role in safeguarding auditory function and preserving quality of life. By adopting proactive measures and minimizing exposure to known risk factors, individuals can reduce the likelihood of developing hearing loss and related conditions.

Protective Strategies for Hearing Health

The old saying that prevention is better than cure will never be out of date. The best way to start a prevention phenomenon is to protect your ears from damage. The following are few strategies for protecting your hearing health:

1. Limiting Exposure to Loud Noise

Prolonged or repeated exposure to loud noises can cause irreversible damage to the delicate structures of the inner ear. To protect against noise-induced hearing loss, individuals should limit exposure to excessively loud environments and use hearing protection, such as earplugs or earmuffs, when necessary.

2. Monitoring Volume Levels

When using personal audio devices, such as smartphones, MP3 players, or headphones, it is important to be mindful of volume levels and avoid listening at excessively high volumes for extended periods. The 60/60 rule—a recommendation to listen at 60% of maximum volume for no more than 60 minutes at a time—can help prevent overexposure to loud sounds.

3. Creating Quiet Spaces

Designating quiet areas in the home, workplace, and recreational settings can provide opportunities for relaxation and minimize exposure to ambient noise. Implementing sound-absorbing materials, such as carpets, curtains, and acoustic panels, can help reduce background noise levels and create a more comfortable environment for individuals with hearing sensitivities.

4. Educating Others

Raising awareness about the importance of hearing protection and safe listening practices can empower individuals to make informed decisions about their auditory health. Encouraging friends, family members, and colleagues to practice responsible hearing habits and seek professional guidance when needed can help promote a culture of hearing wellness within communities.

Promoting Auditory Wellness Across the Lifespan

It is imperative to do the right thing from the start. From childhood to adulthood, promotion of health is sacrosanct in living a healthy long life. Healthy living, therefore, is not an accidental accomplishment. Hence, the following will suffice in making this strong desire in everyone happen.

1. Childhood Development

Early intervention and education are crucial for instilling healthy hearing habits in children and adolescents. Teaching young individuals about the potential risks of noise exposure and the importance of protecting their hearing from a young age can set the foundation for lifelong auditory wellness.

2. Adult Auditory Health

Adults of all ages can benefit from regular hearing screenings, wellness checks, and lifestyle modifications to promote optimal auditory function. Incorporating healthy habits, such as maintaining a balanced diet, staying physically active, managing stress, and avoiding tobacco use, can support overall hearing health and reduce the risk of age-related decline.

3. Senior Wellness

As individuals age, they may experience changes in auditory function and an increased risk of hearing loss. Regular hearing evaluations, communication strategies, and assistive technologies, such as hearing aids and amplification devices, can enhance quality of life and promote social engagement for older adults with hearing impairments.

Authority Citations

1. The Centers for Disease Control and Prevention (CDC) offers resources and guidelines for preventing noise-induced hearing loss and promoting hearing health across the lifespan.

2. The National Institute for Occupational Safety and Health (NIOSH) provides recommendations for protecting workers from occupational noise

exposure and implementing effective hearing conservation programs in the workplace.

By embracing a proactive approach to hearing health and adopting preventive strategies, individuals can mitigate the risk of hearing loss and promote auditory wellness for themselves and future generations. Let us commit to fostering a culture of prevention and empowerment, where every individual has the knowledge and tools to protect their precious gift of hearing.

CHAPTER 6

DIAGNOSIS AND EVALUATION

Diagnosing hearing loss and related auditory disorders requires a comprehensive evaluation by qualified healthcare professionals trained in the assessment and management of auditory function. Through a combination of specialized tests, diagnostic procedures, and patient-centered assessments, healthcare providers can accurately diagnose hearing impairments, identify underlying causes, and develop personalized treatment plans tailored to individual needs.

Comprehensive Audiological Evaluation

A comprehensive audio-logic evaluation serves as the foundation for diagnosing and assessing the extent of hearing loss. This evaluation typically includes the following components:

1. Pure-Tone Audiometry

Pure-tone audiometry involves the presentation of tones at different frequencies and intensities to assess an individual's hearing thresholds across the frequency range. Plotting the results on an audiogram, providing valuable information about the type, degree, and configuration of hearing loss.

2. Speech Audiometry

Speech audiometry evaluates an individual's ability to understand speech in quiet and noisy environments. Various speech tests, including speech recognition thresholds (SRT) and word recognition scores (WRS), assess speech perception abilities and help determine the impact of hearing loss on communication.

3. Tympanometry

Tympanometry measures the mobility of the eardrum and middle ear system by varying air pressure in the ear canal. This test helps identify middle ear abnormalities, such as fluid accumulation, perforations, or tympanic membrane dysfunction, which may contribute to conductive hearing loss.

4. Otoacoustic Emissions (OAEs)

Otoacoustic emissions are sounds generated by the cochlea in response to external stimulation. Its testing assesses cochlear function and can help differentiate between sensorineural and conductive hearing loss.

5. Auditory Brainstem Response (ABR) Testing

ABR testing measures the electrical activity of the auditory nerve and brainstem in response to auditory stimuli. This test is particularly useful for assessing auditory function in infants, young children, and individuals with suspected retro cochlear pathology.

Diagnostic Procedures and Imaging Studies

In cases where there is need for further investigation, there is recommendation of diagnostic procedures and imaging studies to assess the underlying cause of hearing loss or evaluate associated vestibular dysfunction. These may include:

1. Computed Tomography (CT) Scan

CT imaging provides detailed cross-sectional images of the temporal bone and inner ear structures, allowing for the visualization of anatomical abnormalities, such as cochlear malformations, ossicular chain discontinuity, or otosclerosis.

2. Magnetic Resonance Imaging (MRI)

MRI imaging can identify soft tissue abnormalities, vascular lesions, or tumors affecting the auditory and vestibular pathways, including acoustic neuromas, vestibular schwannomas, and other cerebellopontine angle lesions.

Authority Citations

1. The American Academy of Audiology (AAA) sets standards of practice for audiologic evaluation and diagnostic testing, emphasizing the importance of comprehensive assessment and evidence-based interventions.

2. The American Speech-Language-Hearing Association (ASHA) provides guidelines and protocols for audio logic assessment and management, promoting best practices in clinical care and patient-centered decision-making.

By conducting thorough audio logic evaluations and utilizing advanced diagnostic techniques, healthcare providers can accurately diagnose hearing loss, identify underlying pathology, and formulate individualized treatment plans to address the unique needs of each patient. Let us uphold the highest standards of care and professionalism in the pursuit of optimal hearing health for all.

CHAPTER 7

TREATMENT OPTIONS

Addressing hearing loss and related auditory disorders often requires a multifaceted approach that encompasses various treatment modalities tailored to the individual's specific needs, preferences, and degree of impairment. From hearing aids and cochlear implants to assistive listening devices and auditory rehabilitation programs, a range of interventions is available to improve communication, enhance quality of life, and promote auditory wellness.

Hearing Aids

Hearing aids are the most common and widely utilized intervention for managing hearing loss. These sophisticated devices are designed to amplify sound and enhance speech intelligibility for individuals with sensorineural, conductive, or mixed hearing loss. Modern hearing aids are available in various styles, sizes, and technological capabilities, including:

1. Behind-the-Ear (BTE) Hearing Aids

2. In-the-Ear (ITE) Hearing Aids

3. Receiver-in-Canal (RIC) Hearing Aids

4. Completely-in-Canal (CIC) Hearing Aids

5. Invisible-in-Canal (IIC) Hearing Aids

Advancements in digital signal processing, directional microphones, noise reduction algorithms, and wireless connectivity have significantly improved the performance and functionality of hearing aids, allowing users to customize settings, adjust volume levels, and stream audio from compatible devices.

Cochlear Implants

Cochlear implants are surgically implanted devices designed to bypass damaged hair cells in the cochlea and directly stimulate the auditory nerve, providing auditory sensations for individuals with severe to profound sensorineural hearing loss who derive limited benefit from conventional hearing aids.

Cochlear implants consist of external and internal components, including a speech processor, transmitter coil, and electrode array, which work together to convert sound into electrical signals and transmit to the auditory nerve.

Assistive Listening Devices (ALDs)

Assistive listening devices are amplification systems designed to improve signal-to-noise ratio and enhance speech perception in challenging listening environments. ALDs may include personal FM systems, infrared systems, loop systems, and Bluetooth-compatible devices, which transmit audio signals directly to the listener's hearing aids or cochlear implants, reducing background noise and enhancing speech clarity.

Auditory Rehabilitation

Auditory rehabilitation programs encompass a range of therapeutic interventions and communication strategies aimed at optimizing listening skills, enhancing speech perception, and improving overall communication abilities for individuals with hearing loss. These programs may include auditory training, speechreading instruction, communication strategies counseling, and psychosocial support services, tailored to the individual's specific needs and goals.

Authority Citations

1. The American Speech-Language-Hearing Association (ASHA) provides guidelines and

evidence-based recommendations for the selection, fitting, and verification of hearing aids and cochlear implants, emphasizing the importance of comprehensive audiologic assessment and patient-centered care.

2. The Hearing Loss Association of America (HLAA) advocates for access to affordable and effective hearing healthcare services, including hearing aids, assistive listening devices, and communication access programs, to promote inclusion and equal participation for individuals with hearing loss.

By exploring the diverse array of treatment options available and collaborating with audiologists, otolaryngologists, and rehabilitation specialists, individuals with hearing loss can access the support and resources needed to optimize their auditory function, enhance communication abilities, and improve quality of life. Let us embrace a holistic approach to hearing healthcare, where every individual receives compassionate care and personalized interventions tailored to their unique needs and preferences.

CHAPTER 8

LIVING WITH HEARING LOSS

Living with hearing loss presents unique challenges and opportunities for individuals and their loved ones. From navigating everyday communication to managing social interactions and maintaining emotional well-being, embracing strategies for coping and adaptation can empower individuals to lead fulfilling and meaningful lives despite auditory limitations.

Communication Strategies

Effective communication lies at the heart of social interaction and meaningful connection. Individuals with hearing loss can employ various strategies to enhance communication and overcome barriers, including:

1. Open Communication:

Encouraging open dialogue and transparency about hearing needs and preferences with family members, friends, and colleagues fosters mutual understanding and support.

2. Active Listening:

Practicing active listening techniques, such as maintaining eye contact, nodding, and providing verbal feedback, enhances comprehension and facilitates smoother communication exchanges.

3. Clear Speech:

Speaking clearly and at a moderate pace, enunciating words, and minimizing background noise can improve speech intelligibility for individuals with hearing loss.

4. Visual Cues

Utilizing visual cues, such as facial expressions, gestures, and body language, enhances communication effectiveness and provides additional context for understanding.

Assistive Technologies

Advancements in assistive technologies have revolutionized the landscape of auditory accessibility. They offer a wide range of tools and devices designed to improve communication, enhance accessibility, and promote independence for individuals with hearing loss. These may include:

1. Captioned Telephones:

Captioned telephones display real-time captions of spoken conversations, allowing individuals with hearing loss to read along and follow the dialogue.

2. Hearing Loop Systems:

Hearing loop systems transmit audio signals directly to hearing aids equipped with telecoil (T-coil) technology, reducing background noise and improving speech clarity in public venues and meeting spaces.

3. Text-to-Speech Apps:

Text-to-speech apps convert written text into spoken language, providing auditory access to written materials, digital content, and communication platforms.

4. Remote Microphone Systems:

Remote microphone systems capture and amplify speech signals, transmitting them directly to the listener's hearing aids or cochlear implants, enhancing speech perception and reducing listening effort in challenging environments.

Emotional Support and Coping Strategies

Living with hearing loss can evoke a range of emotions, including frustration, isolation, and uncertainty. Seeking emotional support from peers, support groups, and mental health professionals can provide validation, encouragement, and practical coping strategies for navigating the psychosocial aspects of hearing loss.

Authority Citations

1. The Hearing Loss Association of America (HLAA) offers resources, support groups, and advocacy initiatives to empower individuals with hearing loss and promote awareness, acceptance, and inclusion within communities.

2. The American Academy of Audiology (AAA) advocates for comprehensive, patient-centered care that addresses the emotional, social, and psychological aspects of living with hearing loss, in addition to auditory rehabilitation and communication strategies.

By embracing communication strategies, leveraging assistive technologies, and seeking emotional support when needed, individuals with hearing loss can cultivate resilience, enhance quality of life, and foster meaningful connections with others. Let us strive to create inclusive environments where everyone feels valued, heard, and respected, regardless of auditory abilities or limitations.

CHAPTER 9

SUPPORT SYSTEMS

Navigating the complexities of hearing loss requires access to comprehensive support systems and resources that empower individuals to address their unique needs, overcome challenges, and enhance their quality of life. From advocacy organizations and peer support networks to assistive technologies and educational resources, a diverse array of support systems exists to promote awareness, accessibility, and inclusion for individuals with hearing loss and their families.

Advocacy Organizations

Advocacy organizations play a critical role in raising awareness, promoting legislative initiatives, and advocating for the rights and needs of individuals with hearing loss. These organizations provide valuable resources, support services, and community outreach programs to empower individuals and foster positive change within society. Some notable advocacy organizations include:

1. The Hearing Loss Association of America (HLAA)

HLAA is the nation's leading organization representing individuals with hearing loss, offering support groups, educational programs, and advocacy initiatives to promote accessibility, inclusion, and communication access for all.

2. The National Association of the Deaf (NAD)

NAD advocates for the civil rights and linguistic rights of deaf and hard of hearing individuals, providing legal advocacy, policy initiatives, and community empowerment programs to advance equality and justice.

Peer Support Networks

Peer support networks provide individuals with hearing loss and their families with opportunities for connection, validation, and mutual support. These networks facilitate peer mentoring, shared experiences, and emotional encouragement, fostering a sense of belonging and empowerment within the community. Online forums, support groups, and social media platforms offer accessible avenues for individuals to connect with others, seek guidance, and share resources.

Assistive Technologies

Assistive technologies play a pivotal role in enhancing accessibility, communication, and independence for individuals with hearing loss. From amplified telephones and captioned televisions to vibrating alarm clocks and smartphone apps, assistive technologies offer innovative solutions that address a range of auditory needs and preferences.

Organizations such as the Hearing Loss Association of America (HLAA) and the American Speech-Language-Hearing Association (ASHA) provide resources and guidance on selecting and utilizing assistive technologies effectively.

Educational Resources

Educational resources empower individuals with hearing loss and their families to make informed decisions, access relevant information, and learn about available resources and support services. Online platforms, informational websites, and educational materials offer valuable insights into hearing loss, communication strategies, assistive technologies, and advocacy initiatives.

Organizations such as the American Academy of Audiology (AAA) and the National Institute on Deafness and Other Communication Disorders

(NIDCD) provide evidence-based information and resources on hearing health and auditory disorders.

Authority Citations

1. The Hearing Loss Association of America (HLAA) offers a range of support services, advocacy initiatives, and educational resources to empower individuals with hearing loss and promote accessibility and inclusion within society.

2. The American Speech-Language-Hearing Association (ASHA) provides guidelines, resources, and professional support to audiologists, speech-language pathologists, and other healthcare professionals involved in the assessment, diagnosis, and management of hearing loss and related disorders.

By leveraging support systems, advocating for accessibility, and fostering community engagement, individuals with hearing loss can access the resources and support needed to thrive and lead fulfilling lives. Let us work together to create a world where every individual, regardless of auditory abilities, has the opportunity to participate fully, communicate effectively, and achieve their highest potential.

Page **74** of **103**

CHAPTER 10

COMMUNICATION STRATEGIES

Effective communication lies at the heart of meaningful interactions and connections, serving as a cornerstone of social engagement, emotional expression, and personal fulfillment. For individuals with hearing loss, navigating communication challenges requires creativity, patience, and a willingness to explore alternative strategies that enhance understanding and facilitate meaningful dialogue.

Active Listening

Active listening is a foundational skill that fosters mutual understanding and engagement in communication exchanges. Key principles of active listening include:

1. Attentive Presence:

Being present and engaged in the conversation, maintaining eye contact, and demonstrating genuine interest in the speaker's message.

2. Empathetic Understanding:

Seeking to understand the speaker's perspective, acknowledging their feelings and emotions, and validating their experiences without judgment.

3. Reflective Feedback:

Providing verbal and nonverbal feedback, summarizing key points, and asking clarifying questions to ensure accurate interpretation and comprehension.

Clear Communication Strategies

Clear communication strategies enhance clarity and comprehension for individuals with hearing loss, promoting effective dialogue and reducing communication barriers. Some effective strategies include:

1. Speaking Clearly:

Enunciating words, speaking at a moderate pace, and avoiding mumbling or rapid speech patterns enhance speech intelligibility and facilitate understanding.

2. Face-to-Face Communication:

Positioning oneself face-to-face with the listener, minimizing distractions, and ensuring adequate lighting optimize visual cues and facilitate lip-reading and speechreading.

3. Rephrasing and Repetition:

Restating information using different words or phrases, providing context and examples, and repeating key points enhance retention and reinforce understanding.

Visual and Written Communication Tools

Visual and written communication tools augment auditory input and enhance accessibility for individuals with hearing loss. These tools include:

1. Written Notes and Text Messages

Written notes, text messages, and digital communication platforms provide visual cues and supplementary information that support comprehension and retention.

2. Visual Aids and Gestures

Using visual aids, gestures, and facial expressions to convey meaning and emphasize key points enhances clarity and reinforces verbal communication.

3. Captioning and Subtitling

Captioning and subtitling services provide text-based representations of spoken dialogue in various multimedia formats, including television programs, movies, and online videos, improving accessibility and inclusivity for individuals with hearing loss.

Authority Citations

1. The American Speech-Language-Hearing Association (ASHA) provides guidelines, resources, and evidence-based practices for effective communication strategies and auditory rehabilitation techniques.

2. The Hearing Loss Association of America (HLAA) offers support groups, educational programs, and advocacy initiatives that promote awareness, acceptance, and inclusion for individuals with hearing loss and their families.

By embracing effective communication strategies, leveraging visual and written communication tools, and fostering empathy and understanding, individuals with hearing loss can actively participate in conversations, cultivate meaningful relationships, and engage fully in life's experiences. Let us strive to create inclusive environments where, regardless of auditory abilities or limitations, we can hear, value and respect every voice.

CHAPTER 11

ENHANCING QUALITY OF LIFE

Enhancing quality of life for individuals with hearing loss encompasses a holistic approach that addresses physical, emotional, social, and environmental dimensions of well-being. By prioritizing accessibility, inclusivity, and self-care practices, individuals can optimize their overall health and vitality, leading fulfilling and meaningful lives despite auditory challenges.

Physical Health and Well-Being

Maintaining physical health is essential for promoting overall well-being and minimizing the impact of hearing loss on daily functioning. Key components of physical health include:

1. Regular Exercise

Engaging in regular physical activity, such as walking, swimming, or yoga, promotes cardiovascular health, reduces stress levels, and enhances overall vitality.

2. Healthy Diet

Consuming a balanced diet rich in fruits, vegetables, lean proteins, and whole grains provides essential nutrients, supports immune function, and fosters optimal health and wellness.

3. Quality Sleep

Prioritizing adequate sleep hygiene, including consistent sleep schedules, comfortable sleep environments, and relaxation techniques, promotes restorative sleep and enhances cognitive function.

Emotional Resilience and Self-Care

Cultivating emotional resilience and practicing self-care techniques are vital for managing the emotional impact of hearing loss and promoting psychological well-being. Strategies for emotional resilience include:

1. Mindfulness and Meditation

Practicing mindfulness and meditation techniques fosters present-moment awareness, reduces stress levels, and enhances emotional regulation and resilience.

2. Stress Management

Adopting stress management strategies, such as deep breathing exercises, progressive muscle relaxation, and guided imagery, helps alleviate tension and promote relaxation.

3. Seeking Support:

Seeking support from friends, family members, support groups, or mental health professionals provides validation, empathy, and coping strategies for managing emotional challenges associated with hearing loss.

Social Connection and Engagement

Maintaining social connection and engagement is crucial for combating feelings of isolation, fostering meaningful relationships, and promoting a sense of belonging within the community. Strategies for social connection include:

1. Participating in Community Activities

Engaging in community activities, volunteer opportunities, or group hobbies provides opportunities for social interaction, connection, and mutual support.

2. Joining Support Groups

Participating in support groups or online forums for individuals with hearing loss fosters camaraderie, shared experiences, and emotional validation.

3. Developing Communication Skills

Developing effective communication skills and advocating for accessibility and inclusion in social settings empowers individuals with hearing loss to engage fully in social interactions and activities.

Authority Citations

1. The Centers for Disease Control and Prevention (CDC) provides evidence-based resources and guidelines for promoting physical health and wellness, including recommendations for regular exercise, healthy eating, and sleep hygiene.

2. The American Psychological Association (APA) offers resources, tools, and research-based strategies for enhancing emotional resilience,

managing stress, and fostering psychological well-being.

By prioritizing physical health, cultivating emotional resilience, nurturing social connections, and embracing self-care practices, individuals with hearing loss can enhance their quality of life, promote overall well-being, and embrace the richness of life's experiences. Let us celebrate diversity, foster inclusivity, and empower individuals to thrive and flourish, regardless of auditory abilities or limitations.

CHAPTER 12

LOOKING AHEAD

As we conclude our exploration of hearing health and the journey of individuals affected by hearing loss, it is essential to reflect on the progress made, acknowledge the challenges ahead, and envision a future that embraces innovation, accessibility, and inclusion for all.

Advancements in Technology

Technological advancements have revolutionized the landscape of hearing healthcare, offering innovative solutions that enhance accessibility, communication, and quality of life for individuals with hearing loss. From digital hearing aids and cochlear implants to assistive listening devices and communication apps, technology continues to drive progress and expand possibilities for auditory wellness.

Research and Innovation

Ongoing research and innovation play a pivotal role in advancing our understanding of auditory disorders, developing novel treatment modalities, and improving outcomes for individuals with hearing loss. Collaborative efforts among researchers, healthcare professionals, and advocacy organizations drive innovation, promote evidence-based practices, and foster interdisciplinary approaches to hearing healthcare.

Promoting Accessibility and Inclusion

Promoting accessibility and inclusion is essential for ensuring equal participation and opportunities for individuals with hearing loss in all aspects of life. Advocacy initiatives, policy reforms, and community outreach programs play a crucial role in raising awareness, removing barriers, and advocating for the rights and needs of individuals with hearing loss.

Empowering Individuals

Empowering individuals with hearing loss to advocate for themselves, access resources, and participate fully in society is fundamental to promoting self-determination, autonomy, and dignity. By providing education, support, and opportunities for self-advocacy, we can empower individuals to navigate challenges, pursue their aspirations, and live fulfilling lives on their own terms.

Authority Citations

1. The World Health Organization (WHO) provides global leadership in promoting hearing health, raising awareness about the burden of hearing loss, and advocating for accessible and affordable hearing healthcare services.

2. The Hearing Loss Association of America (HLAA) advocates for the rights and needs of individuals with hearing loss, offering support, resources, and advocacy initiatives that promote accessibility, inclusion, and communication access for all.

As we look ahead to the future of hearing health, let us envision a world where every individual, regardless of auditory abilities or limitations, has the opportunity to thrive, connect, and contribute to society. Together, let us continue our journey towards a more inclusive, accessible, and equitable world for all.

<u>CONCLUSION</u>

EMBRACING INNOVATION FOR GLOBAL HEARING HEALTH

In our exploration of hearing health and the challenges faced by individuals affected by hearing loss, one resounding theme emerges – the critical importance of embracing innovation to promote auditory wellness and improve quality of life for millions worldwide. As we reflect on the journey thus far and contemplate the road ahead, it becomes increasingly evident that technological advancements hold the key to unlocking new possibilities and transforming the landscape of hearing healthcare on a global scale.

The Imperative for Improved Technologies

Across continents and cultures, individuals grapple with the profound impact of hearing loss on their daily lives, from communication barriers and social isolation to diminished quality of life and economic disparities. In this context, the imperative for improved technologies becomes clear—a call to action to harness the power of innovation to address unmet needs, bridge existing gaps, and empower individuals to lead fulfilling and meaningful lives.

Advancements in Hearing Devices

Advancements in hearing devices, including digital hearing aids, cochlear implants, and assistive listening technologies, have revolutionized the field of hearing healthcare, offering tailored solutions that enhance accessibility, communication, and overall well-being. From sleek and discreet designs to customizable features and wireless connectivity, modern hearing technologies empower individuals with greater control over their auditory experiences, fostering independence and self-confidence.

The Promise of Telehealth and Remote Monitoring

In an increasingly interconnected world, the promise of telehealth and remote monitoring holds tremendous potential for expanding access to hearing healthcare services, particularly in underserved communities and rural areas where resources may be scarce. Through teleaudiology platforms, individuals can access expert care, receive personalized interventions, and participate in remote consultations, overcoming geographic barriers and reducing disparities in access to care.

Promoting Collaboration and Innovation

Fostering collaboration and innovation is essential for driving progress and catalyzing transformative change in the field of hearing health. By forging partnerships among researchers, healthcare professionals, industry leaders, and advocacy organizations, we can harness collective expertise, leverage technological breakthroughs, and accelerate the pace of discovery, ultimately advancing the frontier of auditory science and enhancing outcomes for individuals with hearing loss worldwide.

A Vision for the Future

As we envision the future of global hearing health, let us aspire to a world where every individual, regardless of auditory abilities or limitations, has the opportunity to thrive, connect, and contribute to society. Let us champion the rights and needs of individuals with hearing loss, advocate for accessible and inclusive environments, and harness the power of innovation to build a brighter, more inclusive future for all.

In closing, let us embrace the transformative potential of technology as a catalyst for change—a beacon of hope that illuminates the path forward towards a world where hearing health is recognized as a fundamental human right, and where innovation serves as a gateway to a life of possibility, connection, and empowerment for individuals around the globe. Together, let us embark on this journey of discovery, resilience, and renewal, as we strive to create a future where everyone can experience the beauty of sound and the richness of human connection, unrestrained by barriers or limitations.